Purpose

Peter E Levy

Published in Australia by Ingram Spark
Design & editing: Sharon Hurst

Acknowledgments

I've seized the chance to incorporate quotes from numerous renowned individuals, honoring their profound insights within the pages of this book. I'd like to dedicate this work to Viktor E. Frankl, whose remarkable life has been a constant source of inspiration for me.

In recognizing the countless pioneers in this fascinating field, I extend my heartfelt salute to them all. It is the collective efforts of both individuals and societies that continually propel us toward a deeper comprehension of the forces that shape our identities. This journey of understanding is an ongoing and evolving process, as it rightly should be.

Peter E Levy

Contents

Introduction

I am not a psychologist but have a keen interest, as a layman, in what makes us do the things we do, and react in the ways that we do. Everyone is different, that's for sure, but as part of the human family, we do have distinguishable features that each of us can recognize and identify with. The concept of purpose is one of those things.

Purpose is deeply personal and can vary from person to person. It is all part of our ongoing journey of self-discovery and growth.

I have found, in my closest relationship, that my wife and I regularly come up with great ideas and concepts. Mostly, however, it is I who does anything about them. That may involve writing a song about the topic we discussed or examining the topic in further detail. Why is that? What drives one person may not drive another. There is no right or wrong to it, but it did raise the questions relating to having a purpose or not.

Purpose also refers to a sense of meaning and direction in one's life. It is the reason we get out of bed in the morning, burning with an enthusiastic desire to do something. So, it can be the reason, or motivation, behind each action we take in that day. As well as the future goals we set ourselves to achieve.

This of course leads us to the actual choices we make, good and bad, that can affect our entire life. Think about it. Those brain neurons that I, and many others, know very little about, can direct us into wonderful and fulfilling ventures just as easily as they can lead us into the darker side of the human experience, where prison walls, both literal and figurative, are the commonplace scenario.

You first must understand the narrative to effect any change that, hopefully, will enhance your life for the better of the community and family that you live with. What will today look like? What could today look like? That's what I am hoping you will discover and investigate within these pages. I have included quotes from famous people to encourage you to realize that we are all on this voyage of discovery simultaneously and that we can learn from, and help, each other in the process.

Meaning and direction

Meaning and direction are two very different but interconnected, concepts that play a significant role in shaping our personal human experience and actions. Let's begin the journey with meaning.

Meaning here refers to the perception that life, or specific experiences, hold significance, value, and purpose. This involves understanding the deeper reasons behind events and circumstances. As we are only able to see and experience things from our own perspective, the meaning will vary from person to person and is totally subjective, even though the same event is being observed by different individuals. We all are going to assign our own interpretations and values to that event, based on our belief system, past experiences, and cultural backgrounds. That is the beauty of the humanity that exists in each of us struggling to make sense of each situation and how we are a part of it.

I'm grateful that my wife and I did a philosophy course some years back, as it opened our eyes to many possibilities that we hadn't considered up to that point. In existential philosophy, for example, the search for meaning is a fundamental aspect of human existence. Philosophers, like Viktor Frankl, emphasize that finding meaning can contribute to mental and emotional well-being, even in challenging situations.

Viktor Frankl was an Austrian neurologist and psychiatrist, as well as being a Holocaust survivor. He is best known for his work on existential analysis and logotherapy, which emphasizes the search for meaning in life as a fundamental human motivation. He survived the horrors of Auschwitz concentration camp by managing to find meaning in the minutiae of his daily life there. The book he wrote as a result of that contains profound insights into the human experience and how to find meaning under even the most ghastly of situations.

I had intended to use many of Viktor Frankl's quotes, but was unable to get the authority from his publisher to do so. Having said that, I do recommend that you do your own research on him and read the book as I feel it will be truly rewarding. (Man's Search for Meaning, Viktor E Frankl, 1959, Washington Square Press)

There were times in my life when I simply

could not understand some of the incidents that were taking place around me. They didn't appear to make any sense at all. After dealing with the stress of unknowing, I put it down to, things happen, and the bigger picture was still a bit blurred for me. And that's alright. We are not expected to understand everything. It is important to realize, that things beyond our immediate comprehension have their own rationale and randomness, and in time we may or may not get to know exactly why those things happened, but we will assign our own rationale and meaning to them.

I now see that all of us need to experience a sense of meaning to things in order to survive the chaos that is ever present in our societies. By doing so, even if it doesn't capture the total accuracy of it, the perceived understanding of it will lead to a greater sense of fulfillment and contentment, as well as providing us with a psychological anchor to fall back on during both positive and difficult times.

The term **direction** refers to having a clear path or purpose that guides one's actions, choices, and goals. It involves setting intentions and making decisions that align with a particular trajectory. When I start a new project, I make sure that I have a framework for setting and pursuing specific goals. This is a very important aspect to keep me focused on what I actually want to achieve, rather than me drifting aimlessly onto any tangent idea that may pop into my head.

It's great to get tangent ideas, provided they fit into your desired direction. So, your choices, ideally, should fall into a process of moving forward rather than sideways. Opportunities will always present themselves as options, and a clear direction pathway should help you to steer clear of those that don't fit your basic goal criteria, and thereby you are less likely to feel lost and uncertain about your next steps.

It is all part of a learning skillset that will enhance your personal growth. Evolving correctly is the aim here. So, when you are totally clear on your direction, it will become a lot easier to persevere and overcome all the many obstacles that may challenge you. It's the long-term long-game that is important on any journey.

Intrinsic motivation

Intrinsic motivation, in this context, refers to the innate desire or internal drive to engage in an activity for its own sake, deriving satisfaction and pleasure from the activity itself. So, it's the fulfillment and achievement of the activity that is the important factor, as against any external reward.

I seem to slip into that mould when writing songs. But, if you think about the process, there is a real pleasure to be derived from it. Certain chord progressions appeal to me at various times and I get pleasure in challenging my initial inspirational thoughts, and trying different progressions to see where it takes me. I'm always conscious of trying not to sound too predictable.

When you feel in control, and a sense of autonomy, there is a satisfaction in whatever success or failure you experience along the route. Your intrinsic motivation will always be higher when it is you who has the freedom to make the choices, rather than being directed to do so from a third party. So, when you have a genuine interest and passion for an activity, you are more likely to hang in there and persist with it simply because it is enjoyable and personally intriguing.

Activities driven by intrinsic motivation, in my case, often lead to sustained engagement and commitment. I would think that anyone is more likely to continue pursuing a task, even when faced with challenges and setbacks, when taking that approach. As I have found, when deep inside my mind on a project, the creative juices have an opportunity to surface and thrive. Concepts of all kinds seem to regularly appear when I do think outside the box and eventually come up with novel solutions.

It doesn't happen all the time but, when presented with a massive task, like writing a movie soundtrack to a defined parameter, my initial reaction is often fear and a big blank page. Once I settle into my rhythm and my own way of doing things, I don't feel so overwhelmed and the task becomes achievable. It allows a certain curiosity of what is possible, mixed with a very positive emotion, like joyousness, which leads to a fulfilling sense of accomplishment and satisfaction when the task is finished.

It is so important to me, and how I live my life itself, to foster these positive emotions. Much better than the reverse. It is all about feeling that you don't require anybody else's assistance. Of course, we all need friends and people around us to assist in the process. No-one is an island. Self-determination, however, brings out autonomy, competence and relatedness which reinforces the elimination of the constant seeking of outside comments or rewards. The activity itself is the reward. When in this state, I have always found my personal growth has increased as I travel down new pathways developing new skills, knowledge and expertise.

> The greatness of a community is most accurately measured by the compassionate actions of its members. *Coretta Scott King*

During this process, time has no meaning as I often go beyond what I think I need, due to the high intensity of my concentration. The biggest problem with all of that is the amount of time I vacate myself from family and friends. My satisfaction of time well spent is soon dampened by my wife who often says to me, "You said it would be an hour and it's now four hours!" But, deep-down, I know that even though I most definitely am at fault and must pay penance for it, I revel in all the newly found potentials gleaned from the total immersion in my project.

So, while intrinsic motivation is such an important driver in fulfilling your purpose, remember that when you are in an adult relationship, it's a mixed bag of balancing your own agenda with being mindful of relationship considerations as well as simply keeping your word.

Personal fulfillment

Personal fulfillment is a unique journey, and what brings fulfillment to one person might not do the same for another. It's important to explore these areas and discover what truly resonates with you and aligns with your values and aspirations. I know that finishing this book will definitely do it for me. Maybe reading it will do it for you.

The unexamined life is not worth living *Socrates*

Having a clear sense of purpose can contribute to personal fulfillment and overall well-being. It provides a sense of satisfaction and contentment. As with meaning and direction, personal fulfillment is also a subjective and multi-faceted concept that can vary greatly from person to person.

I believe the building and nurturing of meaningful relationships is paramount. This involves meaningful connections with friends, family and business partners. I also try to include community members where I live in that list, as it gives me a special bond with people I respect, and a sense of belonging, which is a direct conduit into purpose.

My wife comes first whenever I have any decision, big or small, and she leans on me in the same manner. It's not easy to be always on the same page as each other but we tend to talk it through and reach compromises if we have to. Whatever works. My second-tier support is my friends, and that too is varied as to the level

> Happiness is the highest good, being a realization and perfect practice of virtue, which some can attain, while others have little or none of it. *Aristotle*

of the friendship. You will know which friends will listen and be helpful, rather than just supportive. I see it as a part of my personal growth to ask the right questions and gage the right direction, after weighing up the advice given. It is a skill. All skills require training in some form or another and my suggestion is to keep your friends close, even when you don't require anything more from them than the sound of their voices.

> The purpose of life is not to be happy. It is to be useful, to be honourable, to be compassionate, to have it make some difference that you have lived and lived well. *Ralph Waldo Emerson*

There is a sense of fulfillment to know that you have good friends and not to take them for granted.

> The greatest glory in living, lies not in never falling, but in rising every time we fall.
> *Nelson Mandela*

Another avenue of personal fulfillment is to be supportive of others, even those you don't know that well. Small acts of kindness, volunteering, or mentorship can create a feeling of making a positive impact on your surroundings, and in fact, the world too. That is a win:win all way round in my book. I sometimes let a person with a few items go in front of me at the check-out point at a supermarket. Not a very

> The individual has always had to struggle to keep from being overwhelmed by the tribe. If you try it, you will be lonely often, and sometimes frightened. But no price is too high to pay for the privilege of owning yourself. *Friedrich Nietzsche*

big thing, but it could be something special for the person receiving the kindness. I know I feel good about doing it too, and it doesn't cost anything, and it doesn't take too much from me to do it. If more people did little things for people they don't know, the world would become already a bit brighter. Try it!

> The key to realizing a dream is to focus not on success but on significance, and then even the small steps and little victories along your path will take on greater meaning. *Oprah Winfrey*

A major part of personal fulfillment, for me, is engaging in activities and hobbies that genuinely excite and inspire me. I have always written songs and that task alone is very fulfilling. Of late, I have written novels, plays, filmscripts and attempted more serious ventures, as you can see.

I set a goal and then achieve it. My problem, if you can call it one, is that I have an ongoing yearning to produce something. More like an obsession. Knowing that, I direct my energy, hopefully, into worthwhile activities so as to not waste the small moments of clarity I possess.

There are no rules as to what purpose you see fit to allot yourself, and I do not profess to counsel anyone to follow in what I do. Yours is a personal journey, and only you should decide what is or isn't appropriate. It's really about what satisfies your thirst when the inspirational juices are in full flow.

In helping you to explore your interests, values, and passions (and hence hopefully purpose) reflective practices such as journaling and meditation may also be of help.

> Success is not the key to happiness.
> Happiness is the key to success. If you love
> what you are doing, you will be successful.
> *Albert Schweitzer*

I recommend you to not over-think or over-stress it either. Practise mindfulness and be in the moment, as I do, and just relax into it. Your own creative expression will rise to the surface much better under those conditions, in my experience. I guess it is about honing, and then perfecting, one's personal inner harmony. The rest will take care of itself. If it's meant to be, it will be.

In my readings I have found many quotes beneficial in guiding my own thoughts. After all, we all stand on the shoulders of those who went before. Here are a few favorites:

Happiness is not something ready-made. It comes from your own actions. *Dalai Lama*

To find yourself, think for yourself. *Socrates*

The only way to do great work is to love what you do. *Steve Jobs*

It is not the man who has too little, but the man who craves more, that is poor. *Seneca*

The purpose of our lives is to be happy. *Dalai Lama*

The things you own end up owning you. *Chuck Palahniuk*

The good life is one inspired by love and guided by knowledge. *Bertrand Russell*

To live is the rarest thing in the world. Most people exist, that is all. *Oscar Wilde*

Guiding decisions

Purpose, for me, acts as a guiding compass for making important life decisions. This reflects through my core values. Guiding decisions involves providing advice, information, and insights to help me and others make informed choices that lead to actions that align with my, or their, goals, values, and circumstances.

> The greatest gift you have been given is the freedom to choose your own path.
> *Oprah Winfrey*

I have found that before making any decision, it is important to gather relevant information. By this, I mean, accurate data, facts, opinions, and experiences that are pertinent to the decision I wish to make. There is nothing worse than being vocal over thoughts and ideas that are generally deemed wrong, by the accepted standards the world possesses.

> In any moment of decision, the best thing you can do is the right thing, the next best thing is the wrong thing, and the worst thing you can do is nothing.
> *Theodore Roosevelt*

Misinformation, the scourge of our era, only serves to distract me and I then become side-tracked by irrelevant factors. Get your facts right and quote the source too, so that your choices give you the best chance to succeed in what you ultimately want to achieve.

> The only thing standing between you and your dream is the will to try and the belief that it is actually possible. *Joel Brown*

I often brainstorm ideas with friends to identify potential options as well as to recognise certain discrepancies in my argument. We all come at things from different perspectives and it is wise to assess the advantages and disadvantages before flying headlong in.

> You are the CEO of your own life, and it's up to you to make the tough decisions that will lead you to success. *Unknown*

Think of the consequences and risks at the same time as the benefits. Make sure that each decision you make reflects your core values and not some other value you have inherited along

> Every decision you make is a turning point. *Deepak Chopra*

the way. It's easy to adopt ideas that are not based upon your own values.

We are constantly brainwashed and influenced through all sorts of media and what becomes familiar can easily be mistaken as our own conclusion, when it isn't necessarily. Check everything. The truth is out there if you search for it properly.

There are many resources at your disposal: time, money, man-power, technology, so work through them all, if you can, and be amazed at what you'll find. Sometimes, it pays to go to the experts, because they will bring valuable perspectives that you otherwise would not have even considered. That's why they are leaders in their field.

Try to predict how each decision could impact your future and whether it moves you closer to your desired goals, and where you intend to end up. Then, evaluate the risks associated with each option. Consider how to mitigate or manage these risks to minimize negative impacts. I have often gone with what my gut was saying, especially when I've had prior experience in similar situations.

> The quality of your life is determined by the quality of your decisions. *Robin Sharma*

You don't always have to go the informed routes. I sure don't. I do try to strike the right balance as to whether my decisions will ultimately push me further towards my intended goals. The truth is, a lot of the times it is a trial-and-error arrangement. So long as you don't compromise your integrity and stick within moral principled guidelines, you will generally be well on the road, in the ways you envisioned.

> Your life changes the moment you make a new, congruent, and committed decision.
> *Tony Robbins*

There will always arise non-negotiable options and it is a good idea to list those down early so as not to make the mistake of rushing and then overlooking your own guidelines by using them. Ideas and trade-offs can create tangents of direction and if you keep an eye on the direction they are heading and the possible outcomes, good and bad, future dramas can well be avoided.

> When you have to make a choice and don't make it, that is in itself a choice. *William James*

After the decision is implemented, take time to reflect on the outcomes. What worked well? What could have been done differently? Use these insights to inform future decisions.

> Life is a matter of choices, and every choice you make, makes you. *John C. Maxwell*

The decision-making process can vary based on the complexity of the situation, the level of risk involved, and personal or organizational preferences. It's important to remain adaptable and open to adjusting your approach as needed. You are in command. After all, it's your neck on the line.

> Your decisions determine your destiny.
> *Tony Robbins*
>
> Choices are the hinges of destiny.
> *Edwin Markham*
>
> The decisions we make today create the life we live tomorrow. *Lewis Howes*
>
> The best way to predict your future is to create it. *Abraham Lincoln.*

Resilience and perseverance

> The purpose of life is not to be happy. It is to be useful, to be honourable, to be compassionate, to have it make some difference that you have lived and lived well.
> *Ralph Waldo Emerson*

Resilience and perseverance are two important qualities that play a significant role in anyone's ability to overcome challenges, setbacks, and obstacles. They are closely related, but encompass slightly different aspects of one's psychological and emotional makeup.

A strong sense of purpose can enhance resilience. People with a clear purpose are more likely to persevere and overcome obstacles.

Resilience refers to the ability to bounce back or recover from difficult situations, adversity, trauma, or stress. It involves realizing that the goal-posts have shifted and adapting positively in the face of adversity and maintaining psychological and emotional well-being despite the challenges encountered.

Resilient individuals are not immune to difficulties, but they possess the skills and mindset to navigate through tough times, learn from their experiences, and emerge stronger.

> Your purpose in life is to find your purpose and give your whole heart and soul to it.
> *Buddha*

I have found that resilient people are flexible and adjust their mindset and strategies in response to ever changing circumstances. One of the best examples of that comes from the popular story, *Who Moved my Cheese?* (Dr. Spencer Johnson, 1998)

As a mostly positive person, I tend to focus on solutions rather than dwelling on problems. So, I am always analyzing situations to ascertain why one thing works and another doesn't. I try not to overthink things, as the simpler I can make it, the simpler the solution is, generally. When I put my rational hat on, there is a calmness of non-emotionality. Much easier to think clearly when the emotion is put to one side. Favourite pathways, that are no longer productive, have to be seen for what they are and not for what they used to be. It's a skill that I practise daily in all sorts of situations.

Perseverance, on the other hand, refers to
the determination and persistence to continue
working towards a goal, or whatever it is in front
of you, even when faced with difficulties, failures, or setbacks. It involves the commitment
to a long-term objective and the willingness to
put in sustained effort to achieve it. It's the old
adage of losing the battles to win the war.

Perseverance goes beyond simply bouncing
back; it's about pushing forward regardless of
whatever comes your way. It's about having
grit. Perseverant people maintain their focus
on their goals, even when distractions or challenges arise. They tend to use the setbacks as
stepping stones, learning from failures, using
them to fuel their motivation. I like to think of
my drive as ambition. And, yes, I do have that.

Impact on health

My research suggests that having a purpose in life is associated with better physical and mental health outcomes. I believe it can lower stress levels and improve overall psychological well-being. The impact on health of one's sense of purpose in life is an important topic that has been studied in various fields, including psychology, sociology, and medicine.

Having a strong sense of purpose in life is often associated with better mental health. People with a clear purpose tend to experience lower levels of depression, anxiety, and stress. This sense of direction and meaning can provide a buffer against negative emotions. Viktor Frankl was a great believer in this and quoted several anecdotes from when he was in the concentration camps. One was about just making roll-call in the morning. Having a purpose, albeit small, kept him alive long enough to be finally liberated by The Allies.

> The purpose of life is not to be in control. It's to be connected. *Brené Brown*

Many people with a sense of purpose tend to engage in healthier behaviours. They are more likely to maintain a balanced diet, exercise regularly, and avoid harmful habits like smoking or excessive alcohol consumption. These lifestyle factors can have a positive impact on your physical health. It makes sense, doesn't it? I'm sure there is a link between having a strong sense of purpose and increased longevity.

I also believe that having a reason to get up in the morning and pursuing goals can contribute to a longer and healthier life. Search out like-minds as you will interact better with others who share your passion and energy, and then there will be more emotional support around you when you need it.

I would also suggest that having a purpose in life may be associated with a lower risk of cognitive decline and dementia in later years.

> The soul which has no fixed purpose in life is lost; to be everywhere, is to be nowhere.
> *Michel de Montaigne*

And how about the fact that having a purposeful life might have positive effects on hormonal and physiological systems, potentially influencing factors like inflammation, stress hormone levels, and cardiovascular issues? I'd say, pretty likely.

Contribution to society

Purpose often extends beyond personal benefit and can involve contributing positively to society. Many people, like myself, find purpose through acts of service, volunteering, or pursuing careers that make a difference. Contribution to society and finding purpose in life are deeply interconnected concepts that often lead to a fulfilling and meaningful existence.

> The best way to find yourself is to lose yourself in the service of others. *Mahatma Gandhi*

Contributing to society involves actively participating in actions, initiatives, or endeavours that benefit the well-being and progress of the community, country, or even the world at large. I do this in many ways. The writers' group I run for my local community is just one example.

> We make a living by what we get, but we make a life by what we give. *Winston Churchill*

I would say that giving your time and skills to charitable organizations, community projects, or social causes that align with your values and passions, is the easiest way to slip into this form of contribution. Extremely worthwhile too, as these projects seem to be always under-funded and people involved appreciate what you can bring to the table.

> To give real service, you must add something which cannot be bought or measured with money, and that is sincerity and integrity.
> *Douglas Adams*

If you are of a mind to use this type of activity as a career choice, there are many to choose from. You need look no further than health-care, education, environmental conservation, or social services.

Everyone brings different things to any group or organization, so it is conceivable that you might have new innovations and solutions that address pressing issues and challenges faced by society as a whole. This alone would give you much purpose and self-worth when you enhance the lives of people around you.

> No one is useless in this world who lightens the burdens of another. *Charles Dickens*

You could also try raising awareness about important social, political, or environmental issues and advocating for positive change. It all works hand in hand while you discover your life's purpose, and that involves understanding your values, strengths, passions, and aspirations. It's about recognizing what truly matters to you and aligning your actions with those values. Consider what issues you care deeply about.

> The best way to not feel hopeless is to get up and do something. Don't wait for good things to happen to you. If you go out and make some good things happen, you will fill the world with hope, you will fill yourself with hope. *Barack Obama*

While it is great to try new things and experiment with different methodologies to achieve a uniqueness, the strengths you already possess are maybe a better starting point, if only, that you have proven talents in those areas. Your sense of purpose might evolve over time as you gain new insights and life experiences. Ultimately, by combining your contributions to society with a sense of purpose, this can lead to a deeply fulfilling life, where you're making a positive difference while also finding personal satisfaction.

Remember, that finding purpose is a journey, and it's okay if it takes time to fully understand what you're meant to do. It's also important to note that purpose can come from both small acts of kindness and larger, more ambitious endeavours.

The value of a man resides in what he gives and not in what he is capable of receiving. *Albert Einstein*

You have not lived today until you have done something for someone who can never repay you. *John Bunyan*

Volunteers do not necessarily have the time; they just have the heart. *Elizabeth Andrew*

Service to others is the rent you pay for your room here on Earth. *Muhammad Ali*

Evolution of purpose

Purpose can evolve over time as people experience personal growth, new life stages, and changing circumstances. What brings a sense of purpose in one phase of life might shift in another.

> The purpose of life's evolution is to learn, grow, and contribute in ways that resonate with the essence of our being. *Anonymous*

The concept of "evolution of purpose" can be understood in various contexts, such as an individual's life, societal development, or even in the context of businesses and organizations. At its core, the evolution of purpose refers to how the goals, intentions, or reasons for existence change and develop over time. Nothing stays static for too long and it's easy to slip into routines. While they are good to have, I tend to look beyond the norm, just to see what I'm potentially missing. This works for me.

In the context of biological evolution, the purpose of an organism can be seen as the role it plays in its ecosystem and how its traits contribute to its survival and reproduction.

> The evolution of purpose is a journey of self-discovery, where the destination is not fixed but constantly reshaped by our experiences and aspirations. *Anonymous*

Over generations, organisms can evolve to have different purposes due to changes in environmental conditions and selective pressures. For instance, a trait that initially evolved for one purpose could later serve a different function as the organism's environment changes. I have always thought that the single-cell, from which all life started, is constantly on the evolutionary search for a better way to evolve. Our drive of purpose is also subject to that same search. Just my opinion, and if disproved down the track, so be it.

> The two most important days in your life are the day you are born and the day you find out why. *Mark Twain*

On an individual level, a person's sense of purpose can evolve throughout their life. When we were young, the focus was certainly on personal growth, education, and self-discovery. As we age, the focus shifts towards career, relationships, and contributions to family and society.

Personal experiences, challenges, and accomplishments can reshape one's sense of purpose over time, as well as giving a sense of identity.

> The purpose of evolution is to raise us out of the mud, not have us grovelling in it.
> *Diane Ackerman*

I have worked hard at trying to eliminate many identities that I possess. When I was editor of a national farming magazine, travelling the world with that particular hat on, my identity, or supposed identity, was displayed on my lanyard for all to see. It took me a while to realize I was more than that and none of that, too. Once I sold the magazine business, that previous identity simply disappeared in an instant. With it, my daily sense of purpose totally shifted its focus.

> The greatest achievement of mankind is not in never falling, but in rising again after you fall. *Vince Lombardi*

Societies and civilizations also experience an evolution of purpose. I would imagine that early human societies would have focused on survival and basic needs. As societies advanced, their purpose often expanded to include concepts like governance, culture, education, and more recently, sustainability and global cooperation. They are the noble ones. The darker purposes of war, conquests, power, etc become just as visible and need to be seen for what they are and avoided like the plague.

> The process of discovering our purpose is like peeling the layers of an onion - revealing deeper and more profound truths as we progress. *Anonymous*

Businesses and organizations also undergo an evolution of purpose. A company's purpose might start with creating a specific product or service, but as it grows and adapts to market demands, its purpose could shift to include other values like customer satisfaction, innovation, social responsibility, and environmental sustainability.

> The purpose of life's evolution is to learn, grow, and contribute in ways that resonate with the essence of our being. *Anonymous*

In the realm of technology, the purpose of an invention or innovation can change over time. For example, the internet was initially developed as a means of communication and information sharing for military and academic purposes. However, its purpose has since evolved to encompass global connectivity, e-commerce, social interaction, and more.

> As we evolve, so does our understanding of our purpose, unveiling new dimensions of meaning and fulfillment. *Anonymous*

The evolution of purpose can be seen through various philosophical and existential perspectives. Philosophers and thinkers have explored questions about the meaning of life, the universe, and everything in between. As societies evolve, so do the philosophical questions and the ways people seek meaning and purpose in their lives.

> The path to our destination is not always a straight one. We go down the wrong road, we get lost, we turn back. Maybe it doesn't matter which road we embark on. Maybe what matters is that we embark.
> *Barbara Hall*

Overall, the evolution of purpose is a dynamic and complex concept that involves adaptation, growth, and change over time. It's a reflection of how individuals, societies, organisms, and even concepts. transform to meet new challenges, seize opportunities, and fulfill different needs as the world around them changes.

Individual and collective purpose

Purpose can be both individual and collective. While many people seek personal purpose, communities, organizations, and even entire societies can have collective purposes that drive their actions and aspirations.

> Teamwork is the ability to work together toward a common vision. The ability to direct individual accomplishments toward organizational objectives. It is the fuel that allows common people to attain uncommon results. *Andrew Carnegie*

It's one thing to have individual purpose, but feeling that your actions and efforts can have a positive impact on others or society as a whole, really enhances your sense of purpose. It's a great high to be on, and I revel in every second of it.

> Alone we can do so little; together we can do so much. *Helen Keller*

Collective purpose pertains to groups, communities, organizations, or societies as a whole. It involves shared values, goals, and a common sense of direction that unites members and guides their actions toward a common vision, that may also make a positive impact on society. Collective purpose also shapes the shared identity and culture of any group, reinforcing a sense of unity. It also, hopefully, considers the individual needs and values of all members.

> None of us, including me, ever do great things. But we can all do small things, with great love, and together we can do something wonderful. *Mother Teresa*

Especially in the writing group I am involved with, I have noticed how the collective purpose fosters cooperation, collaboration, and a sense of belonging.

> Individually, we are one drop.
> Together, we are an ocean.
> *Ryunosuke Satoro*

Members of any group generally work together toward a common purpose, leveraging their individual strengths and skills to achieve collective goals. It doesn't work every time when egos and other agendas rear their heads. But it's worth pursuing.

> The power of one, if fearless and focused, is formidable, but the power of many working together is better. *Gloria Macapagal Arroyo*

Confucius and purpose

My intention was to focus, primarily on Western philosophies on this subject. But, as I am currently studying Chinese language through Duolingo, I have chosen to digress here into a small but important part of the ancient Confucian perspective on purpose.

Confucius, also known as Kong Fuzi or Kongzi, was a Chinese philosopher who lived from 551 BCE to 479 BCE. His philosophy, known as Confucianism, emphasized the importance of moral values, social harmony, and ethical conduct in one's life. Central to Confucian thought is the concept of finding purpose and meaning in life through the following key principles.

Ren (仁) Benevolence and Compassion

Confucius believed that the highest moral virtue is ren, often translated as "benevolence" or "humaneness." He taught that individuals should strive to cultivate a sense of empathy and compassion for others. By practising benevolence, people can contribute to the well-being of society and find purpose in promoting kindness and harmony.

Li (礼) Ritual and Propriety

Confucius emphasized the importance of rituals, customs, and proper behaviour (li) in daily life. These rituals and etiquettes serve as a framework for maintaining social order and harmony. By adhering to these norms, individuals can fulfill their roles in society and live purposefully by contributing to a stable and structured community.

Xiao (孝) Filial Piety

Filial piety is the respect and obedience that children should show toward their parents and ancestors. Confucius believed that by fulfilling their duty to their family, individuals not only maintain family harmony but also learn the values and virtues necessary for broader societal roles. Finding purpose in life involves honouring one's family and ancestors.

Yi (义) Righteousness

Confucius stressed the importance of acting with righteousness and moral integrity. Upholding principles of justice and doing what is morally right helps individuals find meaning in their actions and contributes to a just and harmonious society.

Zhi (智) Wisdom and Learning

Confucius was a strong advocate for education and self-improvement. He believed that life-long learning and the pursuit of wisdom were essential for personal growth and achieving a meaningful life. By continually seeking knowledge and self-improvement, individuals can better contribute to their communities and society as a whole.

And as to those individuals whose life purpose is to accrue wealth for the sake of it, Confucius has plenty to say about that. As I understand it: acquiring wealth, for the sake of just accumulating it, is pointless unless it is to be used for the betterment of society.

My conclusion is that Confucius' philosophy of purpose in one's life justifies further examination as there is much to be gained from it.

In summation

Cultivating a sense of purpose is a deeply personal and meaningful journey that involves discovering what truly matters to you and aligning your actions, values, and goals with that discovery.

I'm of the opinion that it's important to define specific goals that align with your passions and values. I have done this technique when arranging the annual *Anthology* for my writers' group. It certainly made the task achievable. Your own goals can be short-term or long-term, and they should give you a sense of direction and motivation.

I know that working towards meaningful goals can provide a real sense of purpose and achievement. Well, it does for me. Why not you, too?

> The purpose of life is not to be in doubt, but to be creative. *E. W. Dijkstra*

I can't stress this enough as to how vital it is to identify your strengths and talents. Leveraging your strengths in your daily activities can lead to a greater sense of accomplishment and purpose. Consider how you can use your unique skills to contribute positively to your own life and the lives of others.

> The heart of human excellence often begins to beat when you discover a pursuit that absorbs you, frees you, challenges you, or gives you a sense of meaning, joy, or passion. *Terry Orlick*

Clarify your core values—the principles and beliefs that guide your decisions and actions. When your activities and choices are in alignment with your values, you'll likely experience a greater sense of authenticity and purpose. Others, around you, will also join the energy and the inclusive contribution will be shared on a higher level.

As I've said earlier, engaging in acts of kindness and helping others can provide a strong sense of purpose. Volunteering, supporting friends and family, or contributing to your community can create a positive impact and foster a feeling of purposefulness.

> Your purpose defines you. Your mission drives you. Your vision pulls you.
> *Matshona Dhliwayo*

Embrace opportunities for learning and growth. Acquiring new knowledge and skills can lead to a deeper understanding of the real world and your place in it, enhancing your overall sense of purpose.

> The purpose of education is to make good human beings with skill and expertise... Enlightened human beings can be created by teachers. *A. P. J. Abdul Kalam*

Challenges and setbacks are natural parts of life. Embracing these challenges as opportunities for growth and learning can help you develop resilience and a stronger sense of purpose. When I was playing squash, back in the day, I learnt little from constantly winning, and a great deal every time I lost.

I still practise mindfulness and self-reflection to stay connected with my inner thoughts and feelings. You also can regularly check in with yourself to ensure that your actions are aligned with your evolving sense of purpose.

> A life of fulfillment is a result of living with purpose. Those who live with purpose have inner peace. *Lolly Daskal*

As you grow and evolve, your sense of purpose may also shift. Be open to re-evaluating your goals and priorities to ensure that they continue to resonate with your current values and aspirations.

It is imperative to reward yourself and take time-out to acknowledge and celebrate your accomplishments, both big and small. Recognizing your progress and successes can reinforce your sense of purpose and motivation.

When you truly get what is happening during the process of purpose and why we do things, great things can await you. Good luck!

www.ingramcontent.com/pod-product-compliance
Lightning Source LLC
Chambersburg PA
CBHW041301040426
42334CB00028BA/3123

HOW TO FIND
YOUR
POINT
OF CONTACT
WITH GOD

by ORAL ROBERTS

A thorough, simple and powerful explanation of using a point of contact to enable you to release your faith toward God by the man who has taught the POINT OF CONTACT to millions.

2015

FAITHFUL EDITIONS, LLC

www.faithfuleditions.com

CONTENTS

1. THE POINT OF CONTACT

Once Jesus asked His disciples, "Where is your faith?" He did not tell them they had no faith. Nor did He say they had never possessed it. He merely wanted to know what they had done with it. The Bible says, "God hath dealt to every man the measure of faith" (Romans 12:3). Faith is not something we have to get; it is the gift of God to us.

I believe that all men have faith, although some may have mislaid it and others do not know how to use it. However, it is not enough to have faith as a potential outreach to God. We must put it into action. Only then can it accomplish the purpose for which God gave it to us.

I was confronted with this problem early in my ministry when people came in front of me for prayer. Some would say, "Brother Roberts, I have all the faith in the world."

But they did not get healed. I wondered about this until God finally showed me the answer. So I used the answer one night when a woman in the prayer line said to me, "Brother Roberts, I have all the faith in the world."

I said, "That's your trouble; you still have it. You must release it. It is not enough to have faith. It must be sent out of your heart. It must be directed to God. As I lay my hands on you and pray for your healing, let my hands be a point of contact to release your faith and send it to God." The woman did and was healed.

God has given a point of contact for the releasing of faith, for the sending of it toward Him. You must create a picture of yourself having faith—having it as though bound within yourself like a captive. Somehow it must be set free and sent to God.

Suppose you have a quarter in your hand. You want to buy a loaf of bread. You are fully capable of buying a loaf of bread because you have the quarter. The storekeeper has the bread waiting. In order for you to get the storekeeper to release the bread, you must release the quarter. You must give it to him or lay it on the counter.

That's a crude illustration, but it helps you

to realize what you must do with your faith. God has salvation for your soul and healing for your body. He has an abundant supply for all your needs, according to His riches in glory by Christ Jesus. He has all things, but you must send your faith to God for what you need.

A point of contact is the means of sending your faith to God. A point of contact is something tangible, something you do, and when you do it you release your faith toward God.

All sources of power have a point of contact through which they can be reached or tapped. You flip a light switch, and what happens? The light comes on. You step on the starter of your automobile and the motor hums. You turn a hydrant and the water comes out. In each case, whatever you do to start the flow of energy becomes your point of contact.

God has given us faith, and He has also shown us how to use our faith through a point of contact. The Bible abounds with examples of men and women of great faith who used a point of contact to release that faith to bring deliverance to themselves and others. David used his slingshot, released his faith and killed Goliath. Moses released his faith as he raised his rod, and the Red Sea rolled back. Elijah let his faith go to God as he struck the water with his mantle, and the waters divided. A woman by faith touched the hem of Jesus' robe and was made whole. Later, we shall examine some of these examples in detail. Here let us consider what a point of contact does when you use it:

First, a point of contact focuses your attention upon God.

Instead of worrying about the future, wondering what's going to happen to you—expecting this to happen or that to happen—you simply turn your mind toward the living God, the Creator of your being. You focus your thoughts, your attention upon Him. You get your mind off your sickness or your sins or your need. You become one with your point of contact. You turn your mind to God, who alone is the answer.

Second, the point of contact sets the time.

If I said, "I'll meet you," and you said, "When?" and I said, "Anytime," and you said, "Where?" and I said, "Anywhere," more than likely we would never meet. But if I said,

"Meet me tomorrow at 2:00 PM at the front entrance of the main post office in your town," then we would have set the time and the place, and we would expect to meet. When you set a time for something to take place, you reach a point of expectation. The Bible teaches you to expect a miracle if you want it to happen.

Third, the use of a point of contact makes all of your believing a definite act of faith.

Your faith is really what you believe. But you can believe without putting what you believe into practice. For example, you can believe that God can save your soul—believe it fully. You can be convinced it is true. You can have faith that God will save your soul. But until you put your belief into action by accepting Jesus, you will not receive salvation. You must turn your mind and heart to Jesus and say, "Yes, Lord, I believe You are the Son of God and can save me from my sins. I accept Your gift of salvation and eternal life."

You can believe that God can heal your body; you can firmly hold to the belief that healing is of God. But until your believing, your faith, becomes a definite, single act, your healing will never come. All your faith must come to a head, a peak, a point, a climax. It must reach a point where suddenly it goes rushing from your heart toward the living God. Then in that moment of released faith, you will feel the power of God come upon your soul, upon your body to set you free.

Fourth, a point of contact is something to which you can hold when the reaction sets in.

Even if you were healed yesterday, I imagine that today the devil tried to make you doubt your healing. Ninety-nine people out of every hundred who get something from God will experience this reaction—the reaction of being opposed by the devil.

The devil will whisper to you, "Look, you have all the symptoms of your old disease. You didn't get healed."

That's when you need to cling to your point of contact and say, "Devil, you will not put that disease or that sin upon me again. I let my faith go to God." You hold to your point of contact and you keep your healing.

Let me give a personal testimony to show what the point of contact meant to me when I was desperately ill with tuberculosis. I didn't call it a "point of contact" at that time because

I had never heard the term used. But now as I look back on it I can see that there was a point of contact. It did for me the four things which we have been discussing.

In 1935, lying in bed with tuberculosis in both lungs, I was getting ready to die. The doctors had given up hope. Then one day my older brother, Elmer, burst into the room and called out, "Oral, come with me. God is going to heal you!" He told about an evangelist who was holding a revival meeting in Ada. He said that when the evangelist laid his hands on the sick and prayed, many were healed.

When Elmer mentioned the laying on of hands, I remembered a Scripture which my parents had taught me: "They shall lay hands on the sick, and they shall recover" (Mark 16:18). These vivid words struck my mind with great force. *I focused my attention on God.* I began to think that if only I could get to that meeting and have the evangelist put his hands on me and pray, God would heal me.

So I agreed to go with Elmer and my parents to the meeting. As we drove the 18 miles in the car Elmer had borrowed, the Scripture kept ringing in my ears and heart. I made up my mind that when the evangelist placed his hands on me and prayed, I would believe God at that moment for my healing. *I set the time and place for my healing.* Although I didn't know what it was at the time, the laying on of hands became my point of contact.

When we arrived, my parents placed me in a rocking chair with pillows at my back because my body was so sore. I waited until my time for prayer came, which was last. As my parents helped me to my feet and held me, the minister's wife put a little drop of olive oil on my forehead. But that was not my point of contact. I kept my eyes on the hands of the evangelist. I watched as he talked. Then he put his hands on my forehead, closed his eyes and began to pray. I heard him commanding the disease to leave my body in the name of Jesus Christ of Nazareth . . . and then I heard no more! Because I had set the time for *that* moment . . . *that* was *my* time!

I didn't know what a point of contact was, but I used one perfectly that night. I was conscious that I was sending all my believing toward God. *My believing became a definite act of faith.* A blinding light came over me. I saw no one for many minutes. I saw nothing but the light that engulfed my whole being. My soul began to sing. A deep fountain of power seemed to break up within the bottom of my being. It came into my lungs and suddenly my lungs were open and I could breathe. I could breathe all the way down without hemorrhaging. My body felt as light as a feather.

When I came to myself, I was on the platform running, jumping and praising God. I knew I was healed, for I had been bedfast for exactly 163 days and had lost the power to walk alone.

About a week later the reaction began to set in. I was back home. I knew I had been healed, but the devil began to whisper to me, "Why are you so weak? Why do you have to rest every afternoon?" I began to wonder about these things, and a cloud of doubt settled on my mind.

One day I was sitting alone in our front yard when my mother walked up behind me and said, "Oral, you're discouraged, aren't you?"

I answered, "Yes, I am. If I am healed, why am I so weak?"

She said, "Well, in the first place you've been in bed so long that you'll need some exercise before your muscles get strong again." And then she told me something which saved my life: "Oral, it may be a year, maybe six months, before you have all your strength back.

The important thing is that the old tuberculosis germs are dead. Now hold on to your healing. It came from God. Do you remember how you felt when the evangelist put his hands on you and prayed?"

"Yes," I said, "I remember." And my mind went back to my point of contact. I could feel the minister's hands again. I could feel the power and glory and the Spirit of God that went through my lungs. *I remembered my point of contact and I stopped doubting.*

That was in the spring. Within 60 days I preached my first sermon and won two souls to Christ. But what would have happened to me if I had not held on to the point of contact through my mother's inspiration when the reaction set in? Probably I would have gone back to bed. Very likely I would have died.

In 1947, when I began my ministry of praying for the healing of the sick through faith in God, God revealed to me the term "point of contact." He showed me how it had worked in my own experience. He also directed me to tell the people how to use a point of contact for the healing of their bodies. I have found over the years that most of the people who are healed, consciously or unconsciously, use a point of contact for the releasing of their faith. They focus their attention on God, set the time and place for their healing, release their faith in one definite act and hold on when the reaction sets in.

2. "IT IS TIME TO GET UP" —LAYING ON OF HANDS

(Mark 5:21-24; 35-43)

The story of Jairus found in the fifth chapter of Mark illustrates the use of the laying on of hands as a point of contact.

Jairus was an outstanding man in Israel. He had a position of respect as a ruler of a Jewish synagogue. Jesus found some of His greatest opposition from church leaders of His day. But Jairus seemed different from most other Jewish rulers of synagogues. He was not so set in his ways as some and seemed to keep an open mind toward Jesus. When trouble came, Jairus turned not to the synagogue but to Jesus.

One day Jairus' beloved daughter became very ill. As a loving father, Jairus did all that he could for her, but she became worse instead of better. Jairus was desperate to know what to do. Then he thought about Jesus. Either Jairus had witnessed some healings of Jesus or had heard about them. So, naturally, Jairus had some thoughts about the power of God to heal. But when his great hour of need came, it was imperative that he should do more than have random thoughts about God's ability to heal. He came face to face with the necessity to reach a conclusion—to make a complete commitment and decision about seeking God's help. As he thought about his child and about the healing power of Jesus, a picture began to take shape in his mind. He could see Jesus standing by the child and laying His hands upon her. This began to be a point of contact to Jairus. He believed that when Jesus laid His hands upon his daughter, she would be healed.

As soon as Jairus decided on his point of contact, he determined to find Jesus. He heard that Jesus was teaching by the Sea of Galilee, so he started in that direction. When he came near, he saw that Jesus was surrounded by a crowd of people. Jairus pushed his way through the crowd and fell at Jesus' feet. (Luke 8:41.) No doubt some people in the crowd were surprised to see this leader of a synagogue kneel at the feet of Jesus. But in his great need, Jairus put aside his pride and did not care what others might think. Jesus was the One who could help his dying daughter. So Jairus knelt there, looked up into Jesus' face and said with great urgency:

"My little daughter lieth at the point of death: I pray thee, come and lay thy hands on her, that she may be healed; and she shall live" (Mark 5:23).

Jesus could feel the urgency of the father's request. He could also sense the conviction in Jairus' heart—his belief that when Jesus put His hands upon the sick girl she would be healed. Jesus knew this was a point of contact for Jairus. God always honors whatever point of contact we set for the releasing of our faith. Jesus could have healed the child by a word. He didn't need to go to her side. But He recognized that the father's faith would not be released without the laying on of hands. So Jesus went with Jairus.

No doubt, Jesus had not finished what He wanted to teach the crowd of people. Probably He had other plans for that day. But He responded to human need which was brought to Him in faith and prayer. We can get God's attention for our healing when we set the time and place and bring our request to Him in faith.

Hardly had Jairus and Jesus begun their journey when messengers came with bad news. They said, "Thy daughter is dead: why troublest thou the Master any further?" (Mark 5:35).

What a shock to the father! Imagine the great fear and despair which must have swept over him. He had put his hope in Jesus and now it seemed that all was lost. But Jesus never fails those who put their faith in Him. He recognized what was happening to Jairus and quickly turned to him with these words of comfort, "Be not afraid, only believe" (Mark 5:36).

Jesus said this for your comfort, too. Do not be frightened. Do not get off course. Hold on to your point of contact. When you hold to your point of contact, your attention will be on Jesus. And a mind filled with Jesus has no room for fear.

Jairus did that. Before fear could take over, he thought of his point of contact. In his mind he could see Jesus by the bedside of his little girl. He could see the hands of Jesus upon her giving her life and strength. So he continued unfalteringly with Jesus to the healing of his daughter.

When they reached the scene, they found weeping and turmoil. Jesus told those assembled that the little girl was not dead, that she was only asleep. The literal translation of His words is, *She is not beyond the reach of faith.*

The people laughed at Jesus. Jairus heard their laughter and saw their looks of scorn. Without his point of contact Jairus might have lost heart. First, the bad news on the way, and now a group of negative people! But Jairus remembered how he had met the first crisis. He had held on to his point of contact and put fear out of his heart. Now he must cleanse his house of fear. Jesus had come this far. Jairus would see that Jesus reached the bedside of the sick child.

So the scorners, the negative believers were put out, even though some of them were probably his personal friends. He went with Jesus to the room where the girl was lying. Jairus watched Jesus reach out His hand and take the hand of the sick girl in His.

This was the moment! This was the time

Jairus had set for the healing of his daughter. He was saying with his mind and heart, "When Jesus lays His hand on her, she will live." Then everything seemed to happen at once. Jairus saw Jesus touch the child. He heard Him say these words, "Talitha cumi," which mean, *Little girl, rise up.* The colloquial meaning of that statement is, *Little Lamb, Honey, I tell you it's time for you to get up.* At that moment Jairus felt his faith rushing out of him to make contact with the healing power of Jesus. And almost at the same instant he saw his beloved daughter stand up and walk. She was healed! She was alive! It had all happened as he had pictured it in his mind. His point of contact had given him courage to go on believing. How thankful he was that he hadn't given up when obstacles came in the way!

It all happened so quickly that at first Jairus wondered if he were still imagining. But when he heard Jesus say, "Give her something to eat," he knew it was true. It was a reality! His daughter had been given back to him to nourish, to care for and to love. Now he would be able to give her more than material nourishment. He could give her spiritual food as well—the joy of knowing Jesus.

Now I know that the raising of the dead is

a rare thing, and there is no indiscriminate raising of the dead taught in the Bible. Likewise, here the journey to healing was undertaken before death claimed the little girl. So our lesson from this is: No matter how extreme the obstacles may seem; no matter how painful the process of healing may appear to be; if you have a point of contact for the releasing of your faith, you can hold on to it and believe for your healing.

Jesus laid His hands upon the little girl and healed her. He laid His hands upon many others, sick in body and in mind—how many we do not know. The heart and compassion of Jesus were in His hands. As He laid His hands upon the people, He identified Himself with their needs. His compassion reached out and found expression in the laying on of His hands. Jesus commanded His disciples to do likewise.

We read in the sixth chapter of Hebrews that the laying on of hands is a doctrine of the Church. Human hands cannot heal, but human hands can be an instrument God uses for healing. And human hands can be the point of contact for your healing.

I believe that the laying on of hands is the highest expression of the Christian faith. It is the man of God stepping outside the pulpit, identifying himself with distressed and suffering people. It is having faith with them for their healing and believing with them. That is why I lay my hands upon the people when I minister to them in prayer.

I know that my hands cannot heal. Only the hands of God can do that. But my hands are my point of contact for releasing my faith for the healing of the people. When I touch someone with my hands in prayer, my heart and my compassion are in my hands. All my faith, all my feeling, all the intensity of my belief in God are poured out in this contact so that everything I feel inside I try to express through the laying on of hands.

At first I thought that everyone I prayed for would be healed if I felt God's presence in my hand. I soon found that this was not true. In most instances, when there was a healing, I was conscious of feeling God's presence in my hand. Yet, there were times when I felt His presence and there was no apparent healing of the person before me. It was then that I understood that I must always carefully explain to the people the value of the use of a point of contact. That is why I have asked you to study the healings in the Bible which illustrate

22

the point of contact. That is why we have examined the story of Jairus to see how he used the laying on of Jesus' hands as his point of contact.

If you use the laying on of my hands as your point of contact, it must be the releasing of your faith as well as my faith to make contact with the healing power of Jesus. Your faith is the key. Your point of contact will help you turn the key and find healing.

3. THE WOMAN'S TOUCH —TOUCHING WITH HANDS AND FAITH

(Mark 5:25-34; Luke 8:43-48)

The name of the woman who touched the hem of Jesus' garment is not known. She was not important enough to have her name recorded in the Bible. I think this is true because God would have us draw courage and inspiration from her story by putting our name where hers could have been. The story of this woman is similar to the story of millions of other people today—believing strongly in medical science, taking advantage of all that good doctors have to offer, spending all they have to get well, and yet still needing healing for their bodies.

This woman had done that. She had an issue of blood for 12 years. Perhaps it was a bleeding cancer. We don't know. But there seemed to be something causing the issue of blood which could not be cured. The Bible says she "had suffered many things of many physicians, and had spent all that she had, and was nothing bettered, but rather grew worse" (Mark 5:26). Evidently the doctors of her day had tried many cures on her. The treatments possibly were painful, but she had suffered them all in an attempt to get well. I am sure the doctors did the best for her they could. But the cure was beyond their skill. The woman spent every penny she had to recover her health. Then, with her money gone, her affliction grew steadily worse.

But somehow she didn't believe that God wanted her to die. She held on to the faith that was in her—that faith that God has dealt to every man and woman. She believed that there must be some way for her to be cured. So she held on to her faith and kept her eyes and ears open. One day some news reached her. There was a Galilean prophet who was going throughout Judea healing the sick and bringing peace to their souls. So remarkable was His power that totally blind eyes had been opened by His touch; the deaf and dumb now heard and spoke; even some of the hopeless cripples were made whole. His name? Jesus of Nazareth.

It was astounding news, but the woman believed it—every word of it. Anyone who can believe in human skill can believe in God's power. For what a man can do partially, God can do completely; and what man cannot do at all, our heavenly Father can do.

This little woman said to herself, "How wonderful this man must be! I can't hope to get near enough to Him for Him to lay His hands on me. I wouldn't have the courage to ask Him to speak the word of healing for me. But, oh, if I can just touch His robe, I know He will make me whole."

And with these words she set her point of contact. If she could but touch His clothes, her faith would be released.

Let us see what her point of contact did for her:

First, the point of contact made her Christ-conscious.

When the woman heard of Jesus and believed to the extent that she could set her point of contact, then Jesus became real to her. He was no longer a name or a symbol or a hope to others. He became *a person* to her—One who could give back her life, her health. Her mind was filled with Him. Long before she saw Him, all other persons faded out of her mind. The doctors faded away. All other ideas faded. All her other plans were laid aside so that her one plan was to make contact with Christ.

The Bible says, "When she had heard of Jesus . . . she said, If I may touch but his clothes, I shall be whole" (Mark 5:27, 28). She saw Him in her mind before she saw Him with her eyes. She made no mental reservations. She was healed in her thinking before she was healed in her body. She saw herself there touching His clothes, feeling His healing virtue and being restored to health—all this before she ever went to Him.

So the woman's point of contact made her

Christ-conscious. It put her mind in the right condition for healing. There was no room for fear because her mind was filled with Christ. Her faith had a chance to act because she knew the source of the healing power and how to turn it on.

Second, her point of contact set the time and place for her healing.

We don't know how long it was after she heard about Jesus before the woman was able to touch Him. But, no doubt, it was soon. She had had enough of suffering. Every day she was getting weaker. Probably as soon as she heard about Jesus and set her point of contact she was on her way to find Him. She didn't think, *Well, someday I'll go find Him,* or, *Someday when He happens to pass me, maybe I'll be able to touch Him.* No, she made it definite! "If *I* may touch but his clothes." She undertook to make the effort. And she knew she must do it soon. Today she at least had enough strength to crawl. Tomorrow she might not have that much strength. So she would set off *now* to find Him.

Some people lose their chance for healing from God because they wait too long. They wait for someone to bring it to them, or they set their time too far in the future. Then they don't have the strength, or they become discouraged during the waiting period. "Now is the day of salvation" (2 Corinthians 6:2). Jesus is near you this minute to bring you healing, to answer your problems and your needs. Be like the little woman and use the strength and the faith you have now.

Third, her point of contact made her faith one definite act of believing.

The woman's point of contact was touching the clothes of Jesus. She wanted to touch His clothes with her hands in order to touch Him with her faith. As she made her way through the crowd she was saying, "If only I can touch his clothes, if only I can touch his clothes!" Her faith cleared a path for her feet and made an opening through the crowd for her.

The crowd may not have moved back for her but she pressed on through. Probably she was on her hands and knees crawling in order to get through the crowd. And then there Jesus was! She reached out a trembling hand and touched the part of His clothes nearest to her —the hem of His garment. She had accomplished her point of contact. At the moment she touched His garment, her faith went rushing out of her to meet the healing power of Christ. It was like touching a live electrical wire. The mighty healing virtue of Christ surged out of Him into her. It went all through her, into every fiber of her being and spent its force against her affliction. In a moment's time, "she felt in her body that she was healed of that plague."

Hundreds of people were around Christ. But the woman was the only one there who touched the power of God. Jesus said, "Who touched me?"

And Peter said, "What do you mean? The whole crowd is touching you."

Jesus said, "Yes, but this was a different touch. I felt healing power go out of me."

Hers was a different touch! She touched Him not as part of the crowd but as an individual. She touched Him knowingly, discriminatingly, purposefully, as a point of contact. She touched His clothes with a specific purpose—to let her faith go out to God. The moment she touched His robe, she believed. Right then! That's the only way to use a point of contact. The virtue of Jesus heals on contact, bringing deliverance from disease and fear and frustration.

There was no healing virtue in the clothes of Jesus, for He said to her, "Thy faith hath made thee whole"—not the touching of His clothes—but her faith. Jesus did not rebuke her for touching His clothes, because He knew they were her point of contact for releasing her faith. God will honor any point of contact that will help us release our faith.

Sometimes people find that touching a prayer cloth will release their faith. There is no healing in the prayer cloth, but touching it is something tangible that serves as a springboard for releasing faith. There is more than one point of contact, for God cannot be limited to any special thing or to any special person.

When Jesus asked, "Who touched me?" the little woman saw that she could not be hidden and came trembling before Him. She told Him why she had touched Him and how she had been healed.

Jesus said, "Daughter, thy faith hath made thee whole; go in peace, and be whole of thy plague."

The woman received even more than she had hoped for. She had felt that her need was physical healing. And she had sought for the need she felt. But He gave her what her whole inner being had been crying for—peace.

By connecting peace with healing, Jesus is saying, "You sought healing for your body. But healing is much more than a physical work. Healing is also a spiritual work. Wholeness is healing for the soul, mind and body. Your faith has made you whole."

Let us remember this: Healing from God is both physical and spiritual. Suppose the woman had found healing from medical science. She would have had healing for her body but not healing with the peace of God in her soul. Her life could not have been changed until she found Jesus. But when she looked to Jesus for her complete healing, her mind became centered in Him. When she touched His clothes, her entire being was filled with His power and she was made whole.

We don't know what this woman did after her healing. But we can be sure that her point of contact gave her something to hold on to. All her life she would be able to see herself crawling through that crowd, touching the hem of Jesus' robe. All her life His words would ring in her ears, "Daughter, thy faith hath made thee whole; go in peace."

4. MASTER KEY TO HEALING—SPEAK THE WORD

(Matthew 8:5-13)

The scene of this dramatic story of a miracle of healing was in Capernaum, the chief city of Galilee and the home of two famous people— a Roman Army captain and Jesus of Nazareth.

The captain was there under orders from Caesar to maintain Roman rule in the city of Capernaum.

Jesus of Nazareth made Capernaum His second home and the headquarters of His ministry on earth. Here He performed some of His mightiest miracles and preached many of His greatest sermons. Here He walked the streets, preaching deliverance by the power of God and healing the sick by His word or by the touch of His hand. He stirred the city.

The Roman Army captain knew when Jesus

entered the city because of His magnetic power over the masses. They thronged to hear Him and to see the wonderful miracles of healing wrought by His hands. At first, the captain was suspicious and hostile. But day after day as he watched Jesus, his feelings changed. He saw that Jesus was not against anybody. He saw Jesus refuse the desire of the people to make Him a king. He saw that Jesus was unselfish and really loved the people. Time after time the captain saw Jesus heal the sick.

When the captain saw the real Jesus, he recognized that He was more than a mere man. The touch of His hand would heal the most hopeless cripple, or a word from His lips would bring life to lost and suffering humanity. His power was above all other power; His authority was above all other authority.

One day the captain's servant became very ill with shaking palsy. The emperor's physician was called, but there was nothing he could do. He said the disease was incurable. The captain was filled with grief for his suffering servant. The Romans considered themselves the master race. They were proud, rude, arrogant—people with no regard for God or man. But this Roman captain loved his servant and was not willing for him to die if there was anything he could do to help him. It dawned on him that Jesus of Nazareth could heal his servant. If he could get in contact with the Prophet, his servant would not die.

The Romans despised the Jews. It was dangerous for a Roman to turn to a Jew. When the captain decided to go to Jesus to ask Him to heal his servant, he knew the risk he was taking. If he was reported to Caesar, he might lose his command or even his life. In any case he was sure to meet with ridicule from his fellow officers and soldiers. The captain was faced with an awful decision and he had to decide quickly because his servant was dying. The captain made up his mind. He decided to go to Jesus, for he believed that Jesus would heal his servant.

While he was on his way to Jesus, the captain realized he was a sinner. All his life Caesar had been his lord and master. Now Caesar could do nothing for him. He needed a new lord and master. When he reached Jesus, the first word he said was, "Lord."

The captain had never called a man lord except Caesar. He had never bowed to any power except Roman power. But now he bowed at the feet of Jesus, looked up into His face and called Him, "Lord."

Jesus instantly responded with His promise to heal the captain's servant. Jesus said, "I will come and heal him" (Matthew 8:7).

This is Jesus—the real Jesus, the unchanging Jesus, the Bible Jesus—responding to suffering humanity. He is saying to us today, "I will come and heal him." That is exactly what He is doing today. He is healing the people when they come to Him in faith.

When Jesus said, "I will come and heal him," the captain replied, "Lord, I am not worthy that thou shouldest come under my roof: but speak the word only, and my servant shall be healed" (Matthew 8:8).

Now we recognize the point of contact which the Roman captain used—the *word* of Jesus. The captain was accustomed to a different kind of power than ordinary men have. Being a military man, he was accustomed to issuing a command or speaking the word. He would say to a soldier, "Do this," and he would do it. His spoken word or command was backed up by the power of Caesar and the Roman Empire.

This was one reason he was able to recognize the power and authority of Jesus. He believed that Jesus had the power and authority of God and that all the power of Heaven and earth were back of His spoken word. Therefore, he didn't request that Jesus come to his house in order to heal his servant. Instead, he said, "Speak the word only, and my servant shall be healed."

The spoken word of Jesus was the point of contact for the captain's faith. It was the point where the captain's faith would make contact with the power of God. It was the specific moment when he would release his faith. The captain was saying, "Your words will set the time. The moment you speak the word, I will expect the miracle."

The point of contact is any point where your faith makes contact with God's power. We have found that Jairus used the laying on of hands to release his faith. He needed the actual physical presence of Jesus with his daughter in order for his faith to be released. The woman with the issue of blood also sought out Jesus. She did not ask Him to lay hands upon her, but she felt the need of some physical contact. But now here is someone who requires no physical contact to release his faith. He asks only for the spoken word of Jesus.

Jesus was amazed. For the first time since He had been on earth, here was a man who truly recognized Jesus' authority and power over sickness. Jesus turned to the crowd and said, "Verily I say unto you, I have not found so great faith, no, not in Israel" (Matthew 8:10).

This is a most significant statement. While He was on earth, Jesus sought faith among His people. He looked for it among the religious leaders and people. At last He found it, but not where people thought it would be. It was in a rough, calloused Roman soldier who came out of his barracks saying, "Lord, you have power above all power. You have authority above all authority. Speak the word only, and my servant shall be healed." Jesus said that was the greatest faith He had ever seen.

Jesus then turned directly to the captain and said, "As thou hast believed, so be it done unto thee" (Matthew 8:13). The Bible states, "And his servant was healed in the selfsame hour." When the captain believed, the healing of his servant began at that moment.

When he believed!—not when he performed some ritual or ceremony, not when he went through some religious form or recited a long prayer, not just through his thinking—but when he believed, when through his point of contact he released his faith!

The captain's believing was completely responsible for Christ's healing his servant. He believed that Jesus was the Lord. He believed that Jesus had power and authority over the sickness and disease in his servant's body. He believed that if only Jesus would speak the word, his servant would be healed. His believing was his faith brought to a climax. His believing did what Jesus told him it would do and what he believed it would do. The servant was healed in the selfsame hour. Jesus, who was there with the army captain, was also with his servant. There is no distance in prayer—no distance in faith—no distance with God.

God tells us in His Word, "I am the Lord that healeth thee" (Exodus 15:26). Do you believe His Word? Do you have the faith of the army captain? Thousands have been healed by making God's Word their point of contact. Perhaps this is the point of contact you need. If you want healing or the answer to some other need, take God's Word and make it your point of contact. Put your hand on the Bible or hold it against your body or just repeat a Scripture. Make yourself one with God's Word. The Book on your body without the words being in your heart is meaningless. But as you speak God's Word or touch the Bible, let it be a point of contact to release your faith. As your faith rushes from you to God, you will find that in the same moment His power rushes into your whole being to meet your need. The words of Christ still have power to those who will become one with His words.

5. JOB'S PRAYER FOR HIS FRIENDS
(Job 42)

The story of Job is one of the most famous stories of the Bible. However, when we think of Job we are most likely to think of his afflictions and the patience with which he bore them. But probably the story of Job would not be in the Bible if its main object were to teach patience in spite of affliction. It is not God's will for us to be afflicted. He wants us to rise above our afflictions and find our way to Him for our healing. How Job did this is the climax of his story and a lesson for those in need of healing today.

It is true that Job was visited by many calamities. His children were violently killed. His property was taken from him. He lost his health. And, finally, his wife turned against him. Job became ill and for days he sat alone upon an ash pile, wishing that he had never been born. Yet, he never accused God or expressed any bitterness toward Him. The Bible says, "In all this did not Job sin with his lips" (Job 2:10). For Job knew what had caused all his troubles. It was fear. The things he had feared had come upon him. Job knew he should blame his troubles on his fear and not upon God. (Job 3:25.)

But Job wanted his friends to understand and to help him. It so happened that his friends thought they knew it all. When they came to see Job, it was not to encourage him to hold on to his faith, or to pray for him. They came to criticize, and criticize they did! They misunderstood the purpose of Job's sickness and suffering and accused him of sinning. They said God had sent the sickness to punish him for his sins. Job knew this wasn't true. His fear had brought on the sickness. God had not sent it to him. At first he endured patiently the criticisms of his friends, but finally he reached the breaking point.

He cried out, "Miserable comforters are ye all" (Job 16:2). Earlier, in a burst of sarcasm, he had said, "No doubt but ye are the people, and wisdom shall die with you" (Job 12:2). What Job said was true. Their attitude was wicked; their words were false. Job also said that they were "all physicians of no value" (Job 13:4). Job was right in what he said, but he was wrong in the way he said it. He became bitter and resentful because he felt he did not deserve the cold criticism of his closest friends. He thought his friends were all wrong. He did not recognize his own self-righteousness.

God looked down upon this scene, and the Bible tells us how His wrath was kindled against these so-called friends of Job. He knew that they had not spoken or done the right thing toward Job. So He spoke to them and commanded them to go to Job for his prayers or He would not forgive them. Then God turned to Job. He knew that His faithful servant was suffering, but He could not excuse Job's burst of passion or his self-righteousness. As Job came into the presence of God, he began to search his own heart. His self-righteousness changed to humility. (Job 42:6.)

Then God dealt with Job and showed him that he must pray for his friends so they could be forgiven. These friends had been weak, had failed to be true friends, and now they themselves were suffering inwardly. God told Job He would forgive Job's friends if Job would pray for them. Job seized upon that prayer as his point of contact.

The Bible says that when Job prayed for his friends, "the Lord turned the captivity of Job" (Job 42:10). God healed him. This was the climax for Job. He had changed his believing. He had become humble. Now he was ready to pray the prayer of forgiveness. WHEN JOB BOWED HIS HEAD AND PRAYED FOR GOD TO FORGIVE HIS FRIENDS, his prayer became his point of contact. He set the time. He made himself one with his point of contact. He put all his faith into one single act of believing—the prayer for his friends. He released his faith and it was then that God healed his body.

It took a lot of courage and love for Job to pray the prayer of forgiveness for the friends who had deeply hurt him. But Job truly loved God and wanted to do the right thing. So Job bowed his aching head and prayed for his friends with all the earnestness he possessed, "Help them, O Lord, and forgive them." When Job prayed for his friends, he forgot himself and put his mind on God. He forgot all the insults which his friends had given him. He thought of the loving-mercy and forgiveness of God.

The purpose of a point of contact is to aid you in releasing your faith to make contact with the power of God. You can see how valuable prayer is as a point of contact. For true prayer is actually getting on the beam on which God is broadcasting. When your radio set is tuned in and the tubes are warmed, at that instant the voice of the broadcaster sounds in your ears. Likewise, when your heart is tuned in on God's way of dealing with people, at that instant you either hear or feel His voice in your heart. It is hard to hear God if the static and clamor of self-righteousness, resentment and bitterness are sounding in your heart. God knew that Job couldn't tune in on Him and find healing until he had stilled the static of resentment. So God showed Job that prayer for his friends was needed. Job used it as a point of contact, released his faith and was healed.

I have prayed for people who have told me that the main cause of their sickness was the bitterness in their hearts. Like Job, they could not focus their attention on God. All they could hear was the noise of their own resentment. By just sitting in our crusade services and without even entering the prayer line, they reached a state of harmony with God and their fellowman and they were healed.

We are told of Job, "When he prayed for his friends . . . the Lord gave Job twice as much as he had before." The last part of Job's life was more abundant than its beginning. We can be sure that Job held on to his point of contact to keep his healing and the many blessings which the Lord bestowed upon him.

6. THE MIRACLE OF NEW FLESH—NAAMAN'S SEVENTH DIP

(2 Kings 5:1-25)

The healing of Naaman, the leper, was mentioned and appreciated by Jesus, Himself, while

44

He was upon the earth. (Luke 4:27.) Jesus commented that there were other lepers in Israel at that time, but only Naaman, the Syrian, received healing. By studying the story of Naaman we can determine some of the reasons he was successful in finding his healing. A point of contact was certainly one of the things which helped him.

Naaman was a famous army general who lived in Syria about 900 years before the birth of Jesus. He was commander in chief of Syria's expeditionary forces. Because of his outstanding military successes, he had been hailed as the national hero. It was shocking news when the general's personal physician found that his chief had leprosy. The disease was common in those days, but it was always dreaded. For leprosy meant *living death*—slow, torturous and isolated suffering. Across the nation, the mournful cry went up, "General Naaman is a leper! Our beloved leader is a leper!"

Some months earlier, General Naaman had made a victorious march across the Bible land of Israel. At that time he had taken captive a little Hebrew maid to be servant to his wife. The girl was familiar with God and His prophets and knew of God's healing power. Seeing the general was a leper, she said to her

45

mistress, "Would God my lord were with the prophet that is in Samaria [Israel]! for he would recover him of his leprosy" (2 Kings 5:3).

When Naaman heard what the maid had said, he was grateful for this hope. He believed the little girl's message and made preparations to leave at once for Israel. Naaman thought that all the effort he needed to put forth for his healing was to make the trip and present himself before the prophet. Then the prophet would do it all. Many people today are like that. All they do is to set a point where they expect someone else to take over, to do their believing for them. They say, "Oh, if only I can get to a crusade, Brother Roberts will heal me."

I can't heal anyone. Only God can heal. I can help you release your faith to make contact with God's healing power. But you yourself must believe. You must have a point of contact for releasing your faith, not a point for handing the job over to me.

Naaman gave all his attention to getting ready for the trip and to making an impression on the prophet so that he would be willing to heal him. General Naaman accepted the girl's witness, but he made a very bad mistake when he went down to the prophet with the wrong attitude. He arrived with great pomp and importance. He brought with him many expensive gifts, and he fully expected an extraordinary reception by the prophet of God. He thought the prophet would rush out and bow down and put his hands over him and do some great thing. Instead, the Prophet Elisha merely sent his servant to say, "Go and wash in Jordan seven times, and thy flesh shall come again to thee, and thou shalt be clean" (2 Kings 5:10).

Elisha was trying to give Naaman a point of contact for the releasing of his faith. But Naaman wasn't ready to accept this point of contact because, to him, it meant *loss of face.* The "loss of face" is a serious problem among people in our world today. Often people miss the message which men of God are trying to give to them, because they are afraid if they do what they are told they will be disgraced or be looked down upon by their friends.

When I was in Formosa and Japan in recent months preaching the gospel and praying for the healing of their sick, I was confronted with this problem time and again. I had heard of the Oriental loss of face but this was my first experience with it. I was in a large auditorium in Taipei, Formosa. The place was packed to the rafters with people, including generals of the army, former ambassadors and various other officials. The first night when I prayed for the people, I put my hands upon them and asked God to heal their bodies. All of a sudden there was a twitter of laughter in the audience. The members of my team and I looked around and wondered what was wrong. What had we done?

After the meeting I went to the missionaries and asked them. They told me that in the Far East you never touch a person with your hands because to them it means a violation of their dignity.

"But Brethren," I said, "this is the Word of God. Christ said, 'They shall lay hands on the sick, and they shall recover.' This is God's way. I cannot change it."

"Well, suppose when you pray for them again you explain that," answered the missionaries.

The next night before I prayed for the dear Chinese people of Formosa I said, "Look, I'm not trying to violate your dignity and cause you loss of face. When I put my hands upon you and pray for the healing of your body, I am identifying myself with you. I am going down into the valley of the shadow of suffering

48

with you. I am your friend and partner, sent here by God. God told me to lay my hands upon you and pray for your healing. In effect, I'm honoring you with all the honor at my command. When I lay my hands upon you and ask God to heal you, I'm honoring you."

I was using two interpreters, but the message got across. After the explanation, instead of disrespectful laughter there were smiles of understanding. Then I prayed for a woman with a goiter. She was a very prominent woman in Formosa, and when God healed the goiter there was a stampede in the crowd. Nearly everybody there wanted me to lay my hands upon them in the name of Christ and pray for them. They then understood what I was doing and why.

The loss of face is a serious thing, even to us here in America. We're afraid someone will laugh at us or will look down upon us. But when we are dealing with God, we must think of what God thinks about us. We must use the point of contact which will best help us release our faith, regardless of how foolish it may seem to others. Like Naaman, we must learn to be humble.

At first General Naaman felt that it would be an insult to go and dip in the Jordan River.

Why, he had better rivers than the muddy Jordan back home! Now, if Elisha had asked him to do something important, that would have been different. I know people like that. They will say, "Brother Roberts, if you will only pray a long prayer for me, I know I'll be healed," or, "If you'll just make sure to call me up on the platform, I know I can release my faith." They are not thinking about the point of contact which will help them focus their attention on God. They are thinking of a point of contact that will focus attention on them.

Naaman was like that. He wanted something fitting to his position. He started to turn away, and then his servants reminded him of the reason he had come to Israel. He hadn't come to get attention. He had come to get healing, and if dipping in the Jordan was the way to get it, then he must do that. Naaman began to understand. He was willing now to accept the point of contact which Elisha had given him. He would get his mind off himself and put it on God. He would be willing to lose face and humble himself.

Let us look at the next scene. Naaman is down at the River Jordan ready to go in. With Elisha's message ringing in his ears, "Go down and wash," he plunges into the muddy, yellow waters of the famous river. He doesn't expect to be cured on the first dip because the prophet has told him to dip seven times. *That sets the time for his healing.* But each 'time he dips, he loses himself. He forgets he is a famous general. He is just a man dying of leprosy. He can do nothing for himself. He must depend upon God. He begins to understand what the prophet meant—absolute humility. Submerging himself in the words of the prophet, releasing his faith to God, he dips once, twice, thrice . . . and the seventh. He is all under. His pride is under, his attitude, his all. *Just this seventh time and it will be done. I know God will heal me,* he thinks.

When he comes up out of the water the seventh time, his faith is released, and he experiences the miracle of new flesh. The Bible says that Naaman's "flesh became again like unto the flesh of a little child." The seventh dip of Naaman helped him to release his faith and make contact with God's healing touch. What a fitting climax—Naaman obeyed the rules of faith and got what he wanted. But he did not forget that God had healed him. His leprosy was gone and God had come into his life. The general made his vows to the true God, that he would worship Him and henceforth would serve no other god.

I am sure that the point of contact helped Naaman keep his healing. If he ever started to look at his flesh for a sign of leprosy, he would remember himself standing there in the Jordan River getting ready to go under for the seventh time. He would remember his joy when he came up and discovered his new flesh. He would know there could not be a mark of leprosy on the flesh which God had restored. His mind would go out to the true God whom he had found in Israel.

7. THE HOLY COMMUNION AS A POINT OF CONTACT

(Matt. 26:26-29;
1 Cor. 11:23-24)

I should like to relate a personal experience to illustrate how the Holy Communion can be used as a point of contact for healing. Shortly before a crusade, I was suffering with a severe cold and a crick in my neck and shoulders. I had tried prayer, the laying on of hands and other points of contact, but somehow my faith wasn't able to break through and touch the healing power of Christ. Perhaps my mind was too much on my aches and pains or I was too concerned about the crusade which was to start in three days. I knew that Jesus would heal me if only I could get close enough to Him. The problem was how to get other concerns out of my mind and concentrate only on Jesus.

Then it was that the Lord reminded me of the Holy Communion. The words, "This do in remembrance of me" (Luke 22:19), kept ringing in my mind and heart. I began to feel that the Holy Communion was the point of contact I needed to release my faith. The Lord directed me to ask a beloved friend to serve the Holy Communion to me. Before I took the sacred emblems, I read the scriptural account of the first Lord's Supper and pictured the scene in my mind. I thought of the real meaning of this observance. Then as I ate of the bread and drank of the cup, I remembered the person of Christ. I could spiritually see Him. I began to be thankful because He died in my place.

And then I discerned His body; I saw that the body of Christ was strong and healthy, that it had no crick in the neck or shoulders, no cold germs, no weakness.

As I thought of this perfect body of Christ, given that I might have abundant life, I could feel my love and faith go rushing out to Him. And at the same time I could feel coming into my body a warmth that welled up in me. It spread from my head to my neck and across my shoulders. Suddenly, I straightened up and I was well. The cold was gone. The crick in my neck and shoulders was gone. I felt fine. I began that crusade with a new force and power.

In all our examples, we have emphasized that there is no healing power in the point of contact itself. The healing comes about through the releasing of faith which makes contact with the healing power of Christ. But the point of contact does help us focus our attention on Christ. It helps to bring Him near so that our faith can reach out and touch Him.

I know of no act greater than the Communion for causing Christ to come personally to you. As a matter of fact, it is the purpose of the Communion for Christ to reveal Himself to you. It is in your act of worship and faith that you discern His body and He is clearly outlined

in your thoughts and vision. I believe the
entire Communion act can be a point of contact for the releasing of your faith if you do
these three things:

First, remember Jesus Christ, the man.

First of all, Jesus said, "Remember me."
He seemed to know that we would tend to forget Him, that we would get our minds upon
other things—the affairs and cares of life. So
He gave us the Holy Communion as something
tangible that would take our minds back to the
Head of the Church, Jesus Christ.

As you take the emblems of the bread and
the cup in your hand, put everything else out
of your mind and think of Jesus Christ, the man.
Let His person fill the screen of your mind,
blotting out all sounds and sights of this world.
See Him as the living, triumphant Son of the
living God. Think of Jesus' being closer to you
than the breath in your nostrils and nearer to
you than your dearest friend. Then you will
know what He meant when He said, "This do
in remembrance of me."

Second, commemorate His death.

Commemorate means *to celebrate*. So many
people make the mistake of being sad when they

take the Holy Communion. There is nothing to be sad about when you take the Holy Communion. Let the emblems in your hand—the bread and the cup—whisper to you, "God loves me. Jesus died in my place. God gave His Son that I might have eternal life."

Give thanks to God that the cross is empty. Jesus Christ has risen from the dead and sits at God's right hand. Look up and rejoice and be thankful that Jesus took your place. Let His supreme sacrifice inspire you to become a living example of God's love.

Third, discern His body.

Jesus said, "Take, eat; this is my body" (Matthew 26:26). Paul said, "Discerning the Lord's body" (1 Corinthians 11:29). The word "discern" means *to grasp the meaning of, to understand.* So Paul was saying, "Grasp the meaning of the body of Jesus Christ." Paul went on to say that many people were sick in the Corinthian Church because they failed to discern the body of Christ.

When you discern the body of Christ, you understand that He had a strong, healthy body. As the bread enters your mouth, it becomes a point of contact. You can hear Jesus say, "This is my body which was given in its fullness to bring deliverance, healing, comfort and encouragement to others—my body which was broken on Calvary for your wholeness." Your faith is released and the health that was in the body of Christ enters your body for your healing and that you might be in health.

The wine which Jesus declared to be His blood represents the life flow that went through His being. The Bible says, "The life is in the blood." His blood was shed for you. And you receive the strength of His blood and His abundant life comes into you as you release your faith through the Holy Communion.

When you eat of the bread and drink of the cup in the Holy Communion, remember Christ. Be thankful and rejoice. Discern His healthy body for your healing and health. Let the whole act of the Holy Communion be a point of contact to set the time for your healing. As you release your faith, you will receive into your very being the life, the strength, the health and power of Jesus Christ, Son of the living God.

8. YOUR FAITH IN ACTION

Things must be *made* to happen. In each instance of healing in the Bible, the person had to do something to get his healing. The woman with the issue of blood got down on her knees and crawled through the crowd to touch the hem of Jesus' garment. Naaman, the leprous general of Syria, did what he had to do, even to bathing in the River Jordan, which he had despised. Jairus had to go and find Jesus and bring Him to the bedside of his daughter in spite of obstacles along the way. The centurion had to forget his pride and position and fall at the feet of Jesus and say, "Lord." Job had to change his attitude and pray for his friends who had wronged him.

There is no deliverance in merely wishing or dreaming that a thing will occur. You find power released through action. You must do certain things. Energies within you have to be released. Your will must become active. Decisions have to be made. Your faith must be sent to God.

I was born and reared in Oklahoma, right in the heart of what is now one of the great oil-producing sections of our country. We did not find oil on our property, but I observed many wells being drilled. I found out that the oil which was being brought from the ground had been there all of the time. The earth contained the oil in abundance, but men had to fashion rigs and drill into the depths of the earth. In one place the men drilled 14,000 feet in order to strike oil. They had to drill deep into the ground and find the oil and release it. They had to cause it to come forth from the earth.

Now this is a very good example that shows how God has placed faith in us and how we are to dig down deep within ourselves to bring it forth. God will not do everything for us. There are some things that He requires us to do for ourselves. The Bible says that faith cometh (that is, it comes out of you as the oil comes out of the ground) when you hear the Word of God and act upon it. Faith will not come forth in any other way. When you release your faith, you will find deliverance. But you will never be able to release your faith unless you are willing to act upon the Word of God.

Once Jesus said to Simon Peter, "Launch out, Simon, into the deep and put out your net for a catch."

Simon said, "Master, we have toiled all the night, and have taken nothing: nevertheless at thy word I will let down the net" (Luke 5:5). From his own standpoint, Simon had no confidence that he would catch any fish. But because the Lord told him to cast the nets, he did so. He had confidence in the word of the Lord and acted upon it. As a result, he caught a big catch of fish.

The promises of God are in His Holy Word, but you can claim them for yourself only if you act upon His Word—if you release your faith as Peter released his net. Only then can you receive the blessings God has for you. Faith which does not dare to take action becomes mere hypocrisy. You must dare to accept the triumph God wants for you. This is your part in the compact between God and you—the active, positive sending of your faith to Him.

How can you put your faith into action?

First, know that God is a good God, wanting you to have the blessings of life.

Second, decide on your point of contact.

Remember, the point of contact itself does not heal, but it sets the time and place for your healing. We have examined a few of the points of contact used in the Bible. In our ministry, many people lay their hands on their radios or television sets when I am praying for the healing of the sick. Many write that they use one of our magazines or books as their point of contact. Act upon the point of contact which God directs you to use, the one that will help you to release your faith.

Third, expect a miracle to happen.

You must expect a miracle if you want it to happen. God is not accidentally handing out miracles. The healing power of God is given on a specific occasion when men and women meet the conditions of God—set the time, reach a point of expectation and wait for God to give His blessing of deliverance. I remember in one of our crusades a little mother who was carrying her child through the prayer line. As I started to pray for the child to be healed of clubfeet, I noticed the woman had a pair of brand-new shoes in her hand. Curious, I said, "Why have you brought the shoes?"

She said, "Brother Roberts, you are my point

of contact. When you lay your hand on my child and pray for him, God is going to heal him. And I'm going to take him over there and sit down and take off these old specially-built shoes and put these brand-new ones on his feet. God is going to straighten my child's feet, and he is going to walk out of here tonight in some brand-new shoes."

Well, it happened just the way that mother expected. God straightened her boy's feet, and he walked out of the meeting in those brand-new shoes. That woman came not only with expectancy but also with expectant faith in Christ.

Fourth, use the faith of others as a guide but never forget that faith is entirely personal.

The faith of others can help you reach a decision to believe. But it is your faith that sets you free. Jesus said, "If *you* can believe." But we have a tendency to say, "Well, Brother Roberts, you believe for me," or, "Mr. Jones, you believe for me." But it doesn't work that way. Others can help you. But you must come to the point where you can release your faith in a single act of believing. Jesus said, "*Thy* faith hath made thee whole."

Fifth, use your key of faith and claim God's promises now.

Your faith can bring the answer to your every need, even at this moment. The healing presence of Jesus of Nazareth is near you now for your complete deliverance. Find your point of contact and let it set the time and the place. You may want to lay your hands on this book or on your Bible. You may want to repeat a Scripture or kneel in prayer. Whatever you do, let your believing be definite and complete. Then hold on to your point of contact and expect a miracle to happen.

"Behold, now is the accepted time" (2 Corinthians 6:2). Start right now to make things happen in your life. Put your faith in action and lay your claim to the promises of God!

A PERSONAL WORD

I have enjoyed preparing this book to help you find your point of contact for the releasing of your faith. If you receive help or need any additional help in prayer, I would be most pleased to hear from you. Thank you and may God give you perfect healing and keep you perfectly whole all the days of your life.

—Oral Roberts

9781943866014